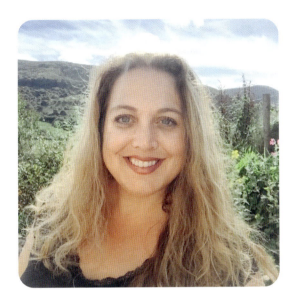

Amanda Porter is a professionally-trained emotional health facilitator and author of the best-selling book on essential oils for emotional healing, Emotions & Essential Oils.

Emotions & Essential Oils was first published in 2012 by Enlighten Healing and sold over half a million copies worldwide, with seven editions in total. Amanda continues to tour and speak internationally on the emotional healing aspects of essential oils.

She is passionate about helping people survive, and then thrive, thanks to emotional healing. She is a mother to two phenomenal children who are her very best teachers and continually inspire her to dig deeper and become more.

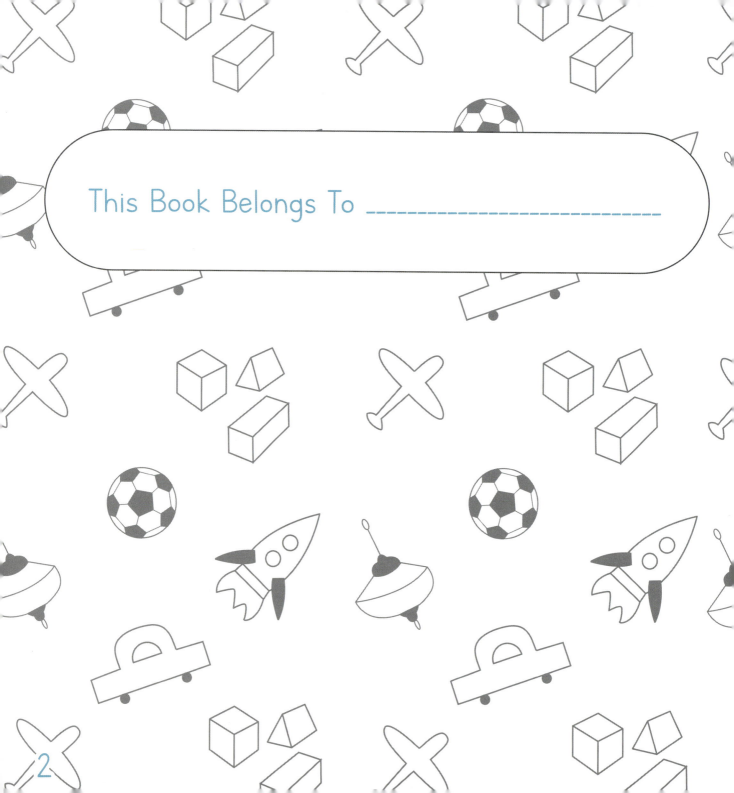

This Book Belongs To _____

Contents

A Message For Caregivers

Growing up can be tough. Everything is being experienced for the first time in childhood and feelings can get very big very quickly. Without the words or insight to be able to express their feelings, children (and adults!) can feel frustrated and misunderstood. Even with the best of intentions, a child's emotional reactions can trigger the unhealed inner-child of the adult and further exacerbate the situation. In order to create healthy emotional terrain and resilient mental health, children need an adult's positive engagement on their emotional journey. How can you do this? You don't need to be an expert! You just need to be willing to talk about a child's emotional experiences and help them learn how to verbalize their feelings in productive ways. Asking how they feel, and supportively listening to their answers, provides a safe space for emotions to be identified and shared. In this book, we partner with essential oils to help you walk through the process in simple, accessible ways. Watch for my "top tips" which provide additional practices to create deeper emotional connection between you and the child you love. I invite you to use this book with a child in your life to help them feel safe expressing themselves, experiencing their full range of emotions, and finding their own positive solutions.

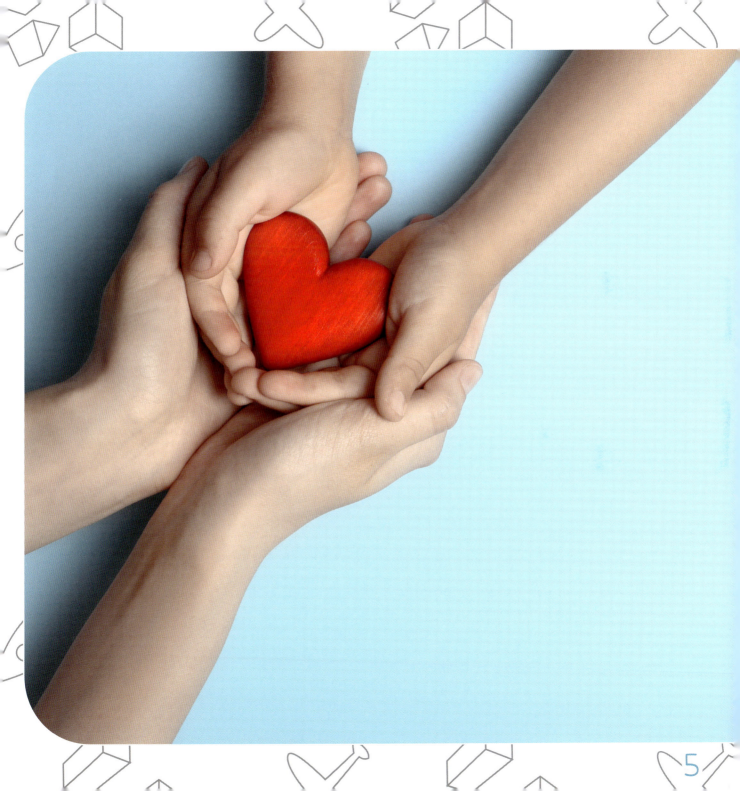

A Message For Children

Dear Children,

Let's become friends with your feelings! This little book helps you learn about emotions and why you may be feeling what you're feeling. You also get to use essential oils (which smell amazing!). Essential oils can help our emotions. Did you know you can also choose how you'd like to feel if you don't like what you're feeling right now? It's true! Only you have power over how you feel inside! And this book will help you learn how you can choose to feel your best. Learning about your emotions and how to respond to them is an important skill to have (more important than learning to ride a bike!). If you begin now, as a child, to listen to the messages from your heart, you will be better and stronger when you're grown up. Really! Sometimes listening to your feelings can seem scary or hard. Just know that a feeling is always scarier when we hide it in the dark and don't let people see it. Once feelings are allowed into the sunshine, to be seen and heard, they lose their scariness and become much easier to handle. So be brave and know that you are strong enough to handle every feeling you have. You can talk about your feelings and still be ok. Promise. You're more incredible than you realize!

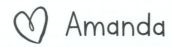 Amanda

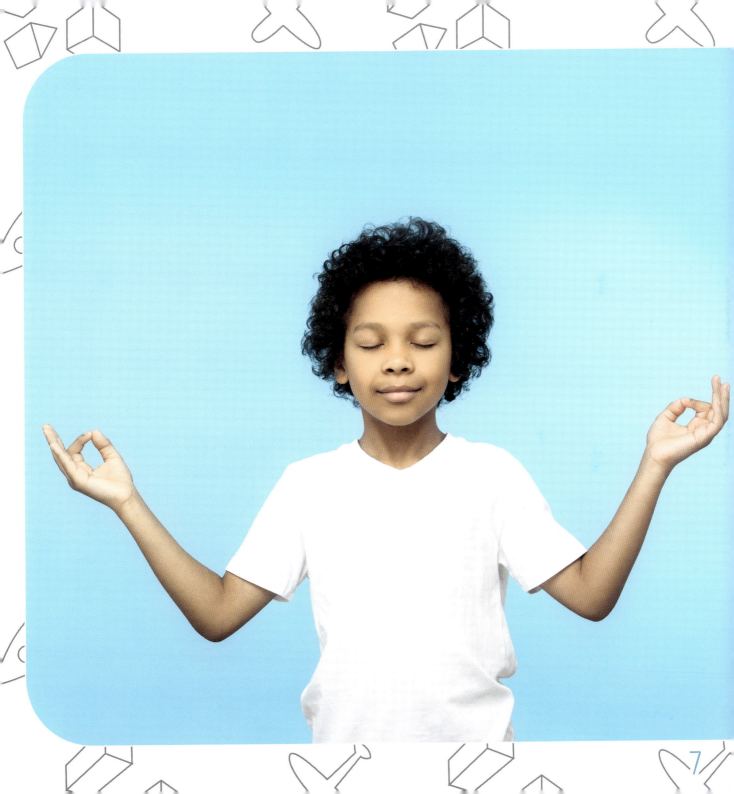

Special Note

Sometimes you may not be sure you're allowed to feel what you feel. Maybe the adults in your life haven't known what to do with their big feelings and so you didn't know what to do either. Did you know that sometimes adults need the good example of a child being brave with their feelings in order for them to feel brave enough to talk about all of their own feelings too? It's true! So know you may be helping people you love by learning these new skills. How nice is that? And the best news of all is that no matter what has happened before you can begin today to become better friends with your feelings and rewrite your emotional story.

And that's a wonderful feeling!

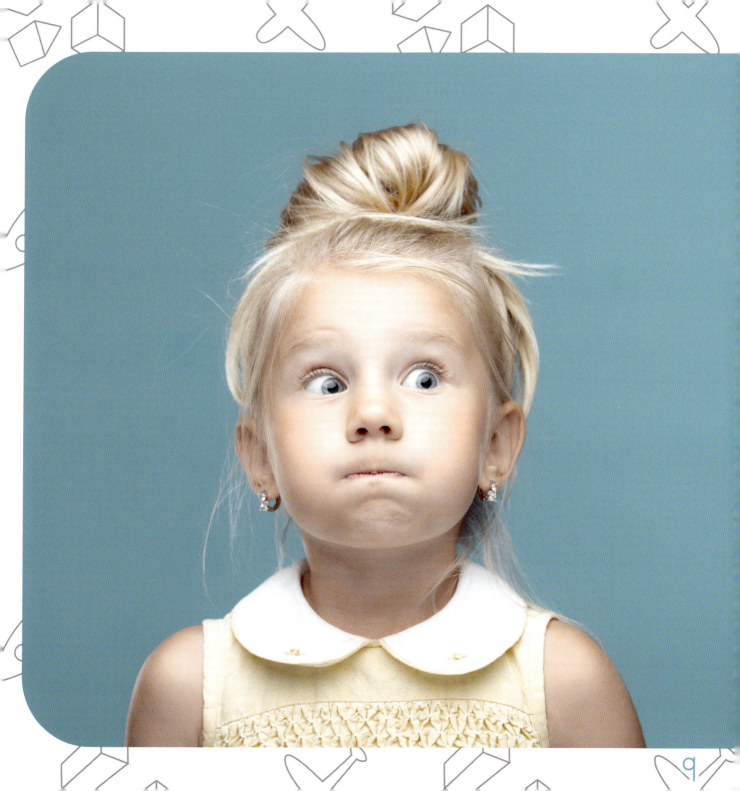

How To Start

If you're a new reader, or not yet reading, start with the emotions pictures and then have an adult help you read through and choose the essential oils that best match how you're feeling right now.

If you're old enough, you can also read through the emotion words under the pictures to identify what you're feeling right now and choose the oil that best matches your feelings.

You can also look at the positive emotions words on the Contents page to quickly choose the emotional states you wish to create. Be sure to ask a trusted adult if you feel stuck or unsure of how you feel. Just talking through feelings goes a long way to helping you feel better.

Let's get started!

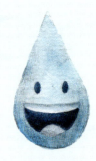

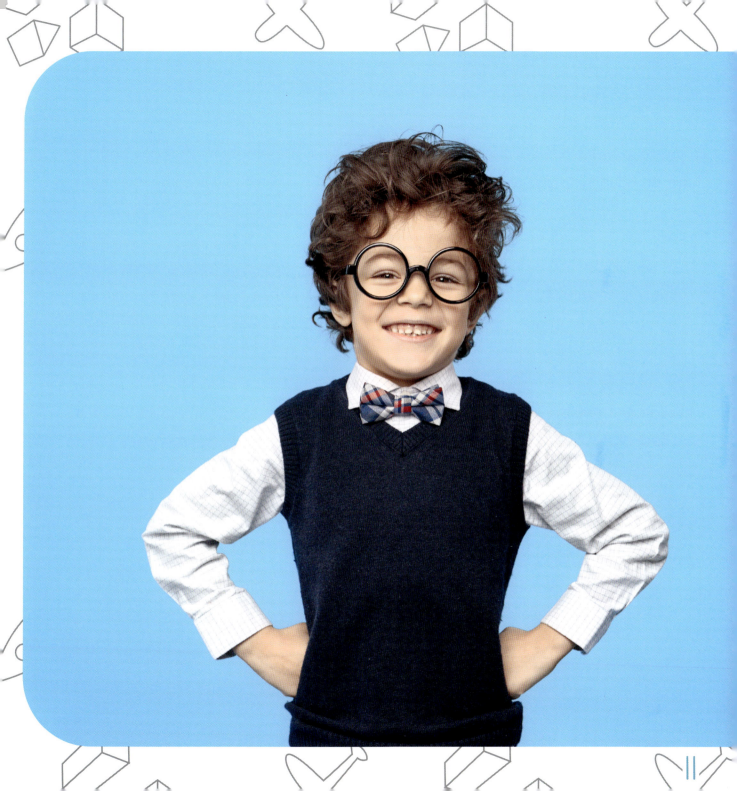

How are you feeling now?

Choose the words or pictures that best match how you feel.

Afraid

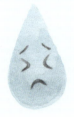

Worried about what might happen

Not wanting to tell the truth

Wanting to hide from something

Best oils:

Brave p. 14
Steady p. 20
Calmer p. 16

Sad

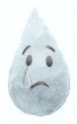

Crying

Wishing things were better

Feeling heavy-hearted

Best oils:

Rescuer p. 18
Stronger p. 22
Thinker p. 26

Angry

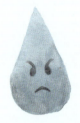

Feeling hot and mad

Wanting to hit or yell

Being impatient with others

Best oils:

Calmer p. 16
Steady p. 20
Tamer p. 24

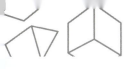

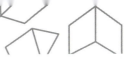

Out Of Control

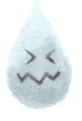

Acting out

Not being able to focus or calm down

Feeling like there's too much for you to do

Best oils:

Calmer p. 16
Steady p. 20
Thinker p. 26

Hurt

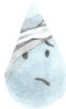

Feeling weak or wounded

Not feeling safe around others

Needing reassurance

Best oils:

Rescuer p. 18
Stronger p. 22

Not Good Enough

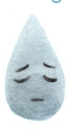

Feeling like something is wrong with you

Trying to be small or go unnoticed

Worried about what others think

Best oils:

Brave p. 14
Tamer p. 24

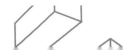
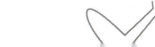

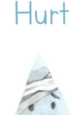

Courageous & Empowered (Brave)

If you need a little help feeling braver, this blend is an empowering choice. Whether it's needing courage to go to the doctor, stand up in front of the class, or to try something new, everyone feels a little unsure or scared at times. Brave essential oil blend is also helpful when you are dealing with other people who are being unkind, hurtful, or not telling the truth. It helps you realize that you are good enough and strong enough to handle these hard situations, and nothing that is said or done to you can ever take away how special you are. Brave blend also reminds you that sometimes you need to speak up when something is wrong. It takes courage to be the one to tell the truth, and Brave essential oil blend will help you face the fear and do it anyway.

Amanda's top tip:

After listening to your child's fears and feelings, tell them how brave they are and how much you believe in them. Affirm your confidence in them, exactly as they are.

How To Use

Roll Brave essential oil blend onto the back of your neck, tummy, or bottoms of your feet (don't forget to breathe in the smell too) before a big moment for that extra bit of courage and confidence you need.

Remember: You can do it!

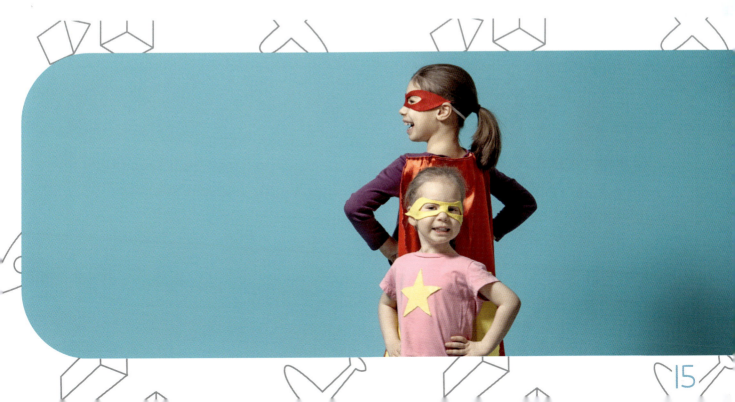

Calm & Collected (Calmer)

When it's time to calm down and rest, this blend is a comforting choice. If you're feeling worried, overwhelmed, or out of control, Calmer essential oil blend is there to reassure you that everything is going to be ok. Sometimes you may feel like life is too big and there are too many things to do and too many people to make happy. If you are feeling this way imagine all of those worried feelings being tied to balloons and see them lifting away from you and floating high into the sky. Once the heavy feelings are gone, feel your body now, and notice how much easier it is for your body to relax. Take a couple of slow, deep breaths and know that you are safe and loved.

Amanda's top tip:

Healthy and loving touch heals. At bedtime, consider giving your child a foot rub while they talk through their feelings and do the balloon visualization.

How To Use

Roll Calmer essential oil blend onto your wrists, back of your neck, or the bottoms of your feet (don't forget to breathe in the smell too) before bedtime or anytime you need to feel a little more calm and settled.

Remember: Everything is going to be alright!

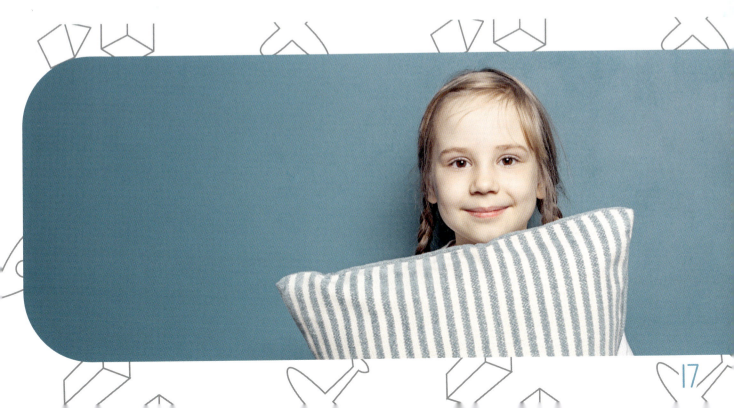

Soothed & Reassured (Rescuer)

If you're hurt or sad, this blend is a soothing choice. When your body is in pain it can make you feel afraid or unhappy. Rescuer essential oil blend is there for you when you need a little extra support to get through life's bumps and bruises. It is also helpful when your heart is hurting. At times your heart just needs a little extra reassurance that it is safe to feel how it's feeling. Everyone needs a good friend to listen to them now and again. So be a good friend to your heart and listen to it when it's hurting. What is it sad about? What does it need? When you listen to your heart, and allow the feelings to come up from deep within you, the pain will lessen and you will feel better. Know that you already have everything within you that you need to heal. Your body is amazing!

Amanda's top tip:

If your child is hurting in any way, have them close their eyes and visualize a beam of light shining brighter and brighter inside of them until it swallows up all their hurts into the light.

How To Use

Roll Rescuer essential oil blend onto the part of the body that is in pain or over your chest (don't forget to breathe in the smell too), to feel soothed and more resilient.

Remember: You are enough!

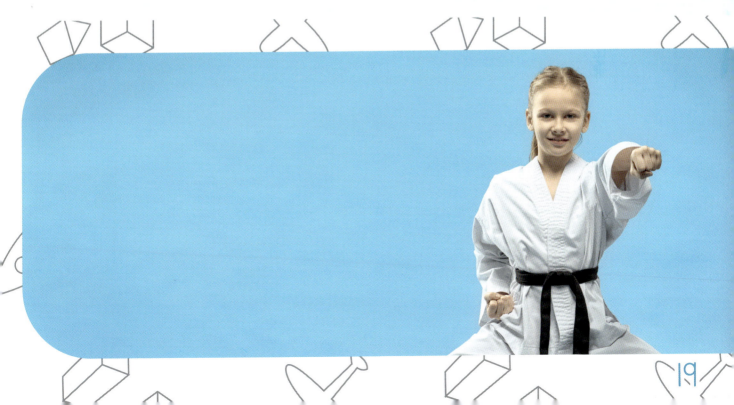

Patient & Grounded (Steady)

If you are worried about the future, or even afraid right now, this blend is a steadying choice. Waiting can be hard and waiting when you're worried is even harder. Instead of letting your thoughts run away with you, focus on what makes you feel calmer or happier. You can sing a favorite song, go for a walk outside, or just take a few slow, calming breaths. If your feelings or actions have been out of control, Steady essential oil blend can help you feel more grounded and self-contained. It gently reassures that everyone makes mistakes and to remember to be kind to yourself and know that you are growing, learning, and changing every day.

Amanda's top tip:

Validate your child's struggles by sharing a time where you made a mistake or felt out of control too. Modeling awareness of your feelings and honesty with your flaws will help them realize they are not alone.

How To Use

Roll Steady essential oil blend onto the bottoms of your feet and legs, and over your chest (don't forget to breathe in the smell too) to feel more stable, patient, and balanced.

Remember: There are no lasting mistakes if you choose to learn from each experience!

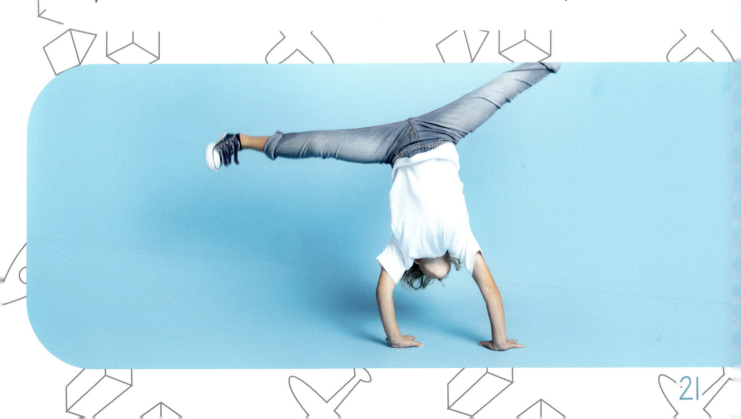

Protected & Safe (Stronger)

When you feel weakened in your body or spirit, this blend is the strongest choice for restoring wellness and vitality. Stronger essential oil blend can help protect you from illness and help you heal if you do get sick. It also helps protect your mind and heart when they feel threatened from the outside. It can be hard to know what to do with other people's big emotions like anger, guilt, or blame. People may even tell you that it is your responsibility to make them feel better when they don't like how they feel. But Stronger blend reminds you that you are not responsible for changing another person's feelings. That is their job and those are their feelings. You can help them by trusting that they are capable of handling their own emotions. This is called having good boundaries. Keeping healthy physical and emotional boundaries with others helps keep you safe and is how you take good care of yourself. This means that you must sometimes let other people be mad at you, or sad because of you, in order to protect yourself. Stronger reminds you that you don't need to be hurt to help others. Good relationships are about being safe and feeling protected. If you are not feeling strong or safe at the moment, imagine a force field of white light going up all around you, shielding and protecting you from everything bad. Then see yourself safe, happy, and healthy on the inside.

How To Use

Roll Stronger essential oil blend onto your arms and chest
(don't forget to breathe in the smell too) to feel stronger, healthier, and protected.

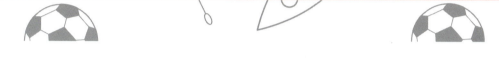

Remember: You are worthy of being safe
and protected!

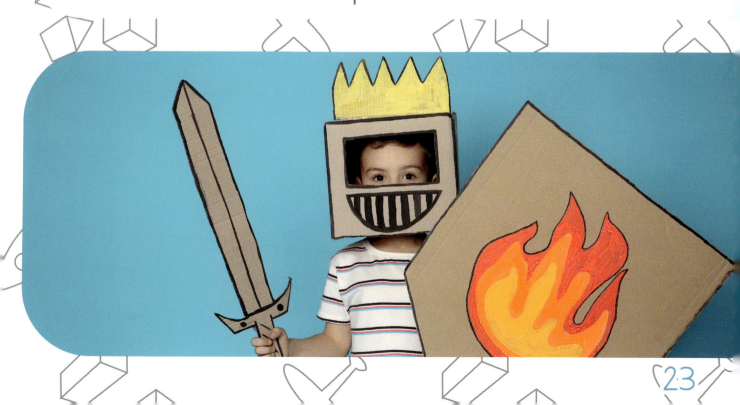

Confident & Relieved (Tamer)

When you're feeling overwhelmed by the big or little things of life, Tamer essential oil blend is a relieving choice. If you are not sure what to do about a situation, or with some of your feelings, it is common to shut down and hide how you feel so you don't get into trouble or feel disapproval from others. When this happens, your feelings get stuck inside and can cause an upset stomach and other symptoms. Tamer blend helps you open up and talk about what's bothering you so you can better integrate and process your life. You will find that your uncomfortable feelings begin to heal once they are shared with someone you trust. If your tummy hurts, imagine a warm yellow liquid filling up your tummy and carrying away anything that hurts or feels stuck, letting it flow and move freely again as it should.

Amanda's top tip:

Stay present and resist the urge to make your child's heavy feelings go away. Practice active listening when a child is sharing their emotions or their reservations, and allow them to express themselves in their own time and in their own way.

How To Use

Roll Tamer essential oil blend onto your tummy and neck
(don't forget to breathe in the smell too) to feel more free, honest, and relieved.

Remember: You can handle your life!

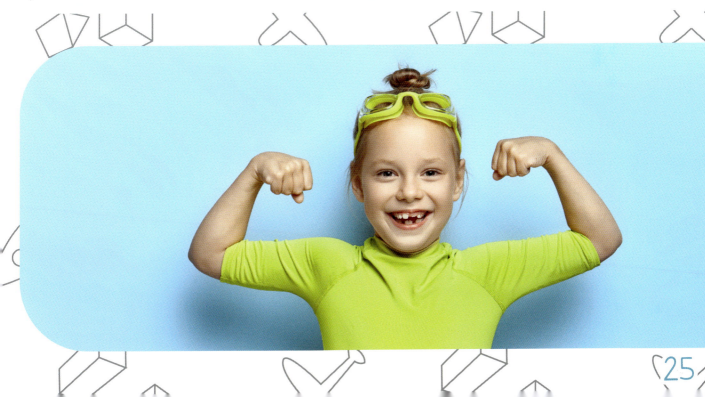

Focused & Clear (Thinker)

When you're feeling confused or distracted Thinker essential oil blend is the clearest choice. It helps to refresh and refocus your mind. It is really helpful for school and when you are trying to study. There is more information all around you and more demand for your attention than you can possibly respond to. Because of this, you must learn to choose what you focus on. It is important to tell the difference between knowledge that helps you and knowledge that hurts you (or others). If something makes you feel uneasy, confused, or like you wouldn't want others to find out about it, then don't do it. Choose things that you know are right and good and you will feel much happier. The decisions and choices you make matter. It is important to also allow your mind enough time to run free and be creative so that it's easier to focus when it's time to.

Amanda's top tip:

Childhood is short and fleeting, and children need unscheduled time to be able to process everything they are learning. Be sure to set aside time each day for your child to engage in free play and unstructured fun.

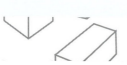

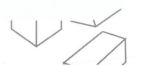

Cover design by Bryce Williamson

Cover photo by © Muhur, sihasakprachum, LUKASZ-NOWAK1

Interior design by KUHN Design Group

Photos on pages 158, 163, and 164 are by Caba. Used with permission.

For bulk, special sales, or ministry purchases, please call 1-800-547-8979.
Email: Customerservice@hhpbooks.com

The Popular Handbook of World Religions
Copyright © 2021 by Daniel J. McCoy
Published by Harvest House Publishers
Eugene, Oregon 97408
www.harvesthousepublishers.com

ISBN 978-0-7369-7909-2 (pbk.)
ISBN 978-0-7369-7910-8 (eBook)

Names: McCoy, Daniel J., editor, author.
Title: The popular handbook of world religions / Daniel J. McCoy, general
    editor.
Description: Eugene, Oregon: Harvest House Publishers, 2020. | Summary:
    "Whether you seek to understand other religions or want to find ways to
    engage with people of another belief system, The Popular Handbook of
    World Religions is a clear and insightful guide to the top belief
    systems globally"— Provided by publisher.
Identifiers: LCCN 2020012318 (print) | LCCN 2020012319 (ebook) | ISBN
    9780736979092 (trade paperback) | ISBN 9780736979108 (ebook)
Subjects: LCSH: Christianity and other religions. | Religions.
Classification: LCC BR127 .P675 2020 (print) | LCC BR127 (ebook) | DDC
    261.2—dc23
LC record available at https://lccn.loc.gov/2020012318
LC ebook record available at https://lccn.loc.gov/2020012319

Printed in the United States of America

21 22 23 24 25 26 27 28 / BP-SK / 10 9 8 7 6 5 4 3 2

How To Use

Roll Thinker essential oil blend onto the back of your neck and your wrists (don't forget to breathe in the smell too) to feel more happy, refreshed, and focused.

Remember: You choose the thoughts today that build your tomorrow!

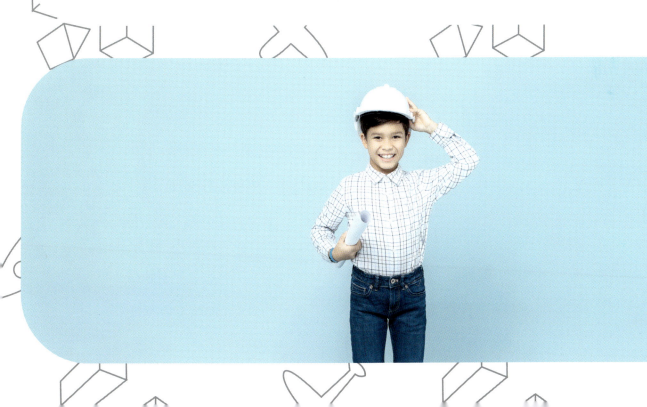

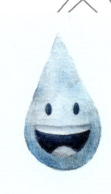

Alternative Kids DIY Blends!

These kids DIY blends were designed by me, Amanda Porter, for my children (and now yours!). Each DIY blend must be diluted with a minimum of 5 ml of carrier oil. I like to make these up in 5 or 10 ml roller bottles so they are pre-diluted and ready to go whenever they're needed.

Courageous & Empowered (Brave)

◊ ◊ ◊ ◊ Wild Orange

◊ Ginger

◊ Cassia or Cinnamon

Clam & Collected (Calmer)

◊ ◊ ◊ R. Chamomile

◊ ◊ Lavender

◊ Cedarwood

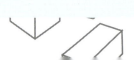
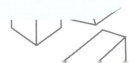